A

JOURNEY TOWARDS

UNDERSTANDING

AND

PREVENTION

OF

HEPATITIS B

By

Olivia S. Rivers

"Outsmarting the Silent Assassin:
Coping with Hepatitis B"

COPYRIGHT PAGE

This book, titled "A Journey Towards Understanding and Prevention of Hepatitis B," is a work that provides professional advice. The information provided in this book is based on the author's research and personal experience and should not be considered a substitute for consulting with a healthcare professional. The author and publisher disclaim any liability arising from the use of the information contained in this book.

For permissions requests, please contact the publisher at [amazone.com].

TABLE OF CONTENTS

CHAPTER ONE

1.0 Introduction to Hepatitis B

Once upon a time, in a small town called Oakwood, there lived a young woman named Sarah. Sarah had been diagnosed with hepatitis B, a chronic liver infection, when she was just a teenager. Despite the challenges she faced, Sarah never let her condition define her. She was determined to live a fulfilling life and make a positive impact on those around her. Sarah's journey with hepatitis B was not an easy one. She experienced periods of fatigue, jaundice, and occasional flare-ups, which often left her feeling frustrated and discouraged. However, she relied on her strong support system, including her family, friends, and healthcare professionals, to help her through the tough times.

As Sarah grew older, she discovered her passion for raising awareness about hepatitis B and supporting others who were also living with this condition. She joined a local support group where she met individuals from different walks of life, all connected by their experiences with hepatitis B. Together, they organized educational campaigns and fundraising events and shared their stories to spread awareness and eliminate the stigma surrounding the disease. Sarah's dedication and hard work did not go unnoticed. She caught the attention of a national hepatitis B advocacy organization, which invited her to become a spokesperson for their cause. With this platform, Sarah was able to reach a wider audience and make an even greater impact. She traveled to different cities, participated in conferences, and shared her personal journey to inspire others living with hepatitis B. Over time, Sarah's efforts began to yield results.

The Hepatitis B Virus (HBV)

The hepatitis B virus (HBV) is the source of hepatitis B, a viral infection that damages the liver. It is among the most widespread and dangerous viral diseases in the world. Hepatitis B can have a serious negative influence on a person's health and quality of life and can cause both acute and chronic liver damage. Contact with an infected person's blood or other bodily fluids is the main way that the virus is spread. It can be transmitted in a number of ways, including unprotected sexual contact, sharing syringes or needles, transfer from mother to child during childbirth, and direct contact with the blood or open sores of an infected individual.

1.2 History and Symptoms of Hepatitis B

It is essential to comprehend the hepatitis B history and symptoms in order to prevent, diagnose, and treat the disease. Although the cause of hepatitis B is still up for debate in science, the illness has long been recognized as different. Hepatitis B instances were first recorded more than 4,500 years ago in ancient China, when historical records mentioned an illness that sounded like hepatitis. But Dr. Baruch Blumberg didn't identify and isolate the hepatitis B virus until the 1960s, which is when the vaccine against the virus was created.

Symptoms

Hepatitis B symptoms can range in severity from moderate to severe and are not always evident right away. While some people may show no symptoms at all, others may have a variety of symptoms that point to liver failure. *The following are typical signs and symptoms of hepatitis B:*

1. Fatigue: One of the most prevalent symptoms of hepatitis B is feeling extremely weary or low in energy. This exhaustion may be ongoing and interfere with day-to-day tasks.

2. Jaundice: The yellowing of the skin and eyes is the hallmark of jaundice. It happens when

bilirubin, a yellow pigment created by the breakdown of red blood cells, cannot be processed by the liver.

1.3 The Global Impact of Hepatitis B: A Silent Epidemic

The hepatitis B virus (HBV) is the source of hepatitis B, a viral infection that damages the liver. With almost 257 million chronically infected individuals worldwide, it is a global health concern. The effects of this silent epidemic on people, communities, and healthcare systems are significant. We will discuss the difficulties in diagnosing, treating, and preventing hepatitis B while also examining the disease's worldwide effects. *The global impact of hepatitis B is significant, with several key points highlighting its importance:*

Prevalence: Hepatitis B is one of the most common viral infections globally. According to the World Health Organization (WHO), an estimated 257 million people were living with chronic hepatitis B infection in 2019. This accounts for around 3.5% of the global population.

Regional Variations: The burden of hepatitis B is not evenly distributed across the globe. It is particularly prevalent in Africa, the Western Pacific region, and parts of Asia, where rates of infection are much higher than the global average. In these regions, the virus is often transmitted from mother to child during childbirth or through other modes of transmission, such as unsafe medical procedures or injection drug use.

Impact on Health: Hepatitis B can lead to severe liver disease, including cirrhosis, liver cancer, and liver failure. It is a leading cause of liver-related morbidity and mortality worldwide. According to the WHO, approximately 887,000 deaths occurred in 2019 due to complications related to hepatitis B, including liver cancer and cirrhosis.

Economic Burden: The global economic burden of hepatitis B is substantial. This includes the costs associated with healthcare services such as diagnosis, treatment, and managing the complications that may arise from the disease. The cost of diagnosis involves testing individuals for hepatitis B, which can include blood tests and other diagnostic procedures. Treatment costs usually involve antiviral medications and other therapies that are necessary to manage the disease and minimize its impact on the patient's health. Additionally, managing the complications of hepatitis B can also add to the economic burden. Complications can include liver cirrhosis, liver cancer, and other liver-related diseases, which may require specialized care, hospitalization, and even liver transplants.

These costs not only affect individuals who are directly impacted by hepatitis B but also burden healthcare systems and societies as a whole. They can strain healthcare budgets, increase insurance premiums, and place financial stress on individuals and families. Understanding the economic burden of hepatitis B is crucial for policymakers, healthcare providers, and researchers to develop strategies and interventions to mitigate the costs associated with this disease and improve overall healthcare outcomes.

1.4 Prevention and Control of Hepatitis B Require a Comprehensive Approach

Certainly! Vaccination is indeed a key preventive measure in healthcare. It involves the administration of vaccines, which are substances containing weakened or inactivated pathogens or parts of pathogens. By introducing these substances into the body, vaccines stimulate the immune system to recognize and combat specific diseases. Vaccines have undergone rigorous testing and have been proven to be highly effective in preventing new infections. They work by triggering the production of antibodies, which are proteins that help the immune system recognize and fight off specific pathogens. Additionally, vaccines also stimulate the production of memory cells, which "remember" the pathogen so that the body can mount a faster and stronger defense if exposed to the same pathogen in the future.

Vaccination has played a crucial role in the eradication or significant reduction of many infectious diseases, such as smallpox, polio, measles, and diphtheria. It has saved countless lives and prevented the spread of these diseases within communities and populations. Vaccination not only protects the individual receiving the vaccine but also helps to create herd immunity, preventing the rapid spread of diseases within a population. It is important to note that vaccines are thoroughly tested for safety and efficacy before being approved for public use. The benefits of vaccination far outweigh the risks, which are generally minimal and rare. Vaccination is a crucial tool in public health, and it continues to be recommended and promoted as a highly effective preventive measure against new infections.

1.5 Global Strategies for Hepatitis B Control

Hepatitis B is a significant global health issue, affecting millions of people worldwide. It is a viral infection that can lead to chronic liver disease, liver cirrhosis, and even liver cancer. In light of its socio-economic impact, various global strategies have been implemented to control the spread of hepatitis B and reduce its burden on affected populations. *Below are* some essential strategies that have been employed to combat hepatitis B on a global scale.

1. **Universal Vaccination:** One of the key strategies for hepatitis B control is the implementation of universal vaccination programs. Vaccination has proven to be highly effective in preventing new infections. By integrating hepatitis B vaccines into routine immunization schedules, countries can provide long-term protection to their populations, especially infants and high-risk groups such as healthcare workers and people living with HIV.

2. **Increased Awareness and Education:** Raising awareness about hepatitis B is crucial for prevention and control. Public education campaigns aim to promote knowledge about transmission routes, risk

factors, and the importance of vaccination. By educating communities, healthcare professionals, and policymakers, we can reduce stigma, encourage early detection, and promote adherence to treatment guidelines.

1.3 Improved screening and diagnosis:

Identifying individuals infected with hepatitis B is essential for timely intervention and prevention of transmission. Global strategies focus on improving access to affordable and accurate diagnostic tests, such as hepatitis B surface antigen (HBsAg) tests. Scaling up screening programs,

1.6 Social and Economic Impact

There is a substantial social and economic consequence of hepatitis B. People infected with the virus frequently experience discrimination and stigma, which lowers their quality of life and causes them to become socially isolated. Furthermore, because hepatitis B can cause persistent fatigue and other symptoms that impair one's capacity to work, it can have a negative impact on productivity. Over 250 million people globally are thought to have a chronic hepatitis B infection, which makes it a serious public health issue. The possible long-term effects of hepatitis B are among its most concerning features. Hepatitis B can cause liver cirrhosis, liver cancer, and even death if it is not treated or misdiagnosed. Indeed, liver illness associated with hepatitis B is thought to be the cause of about 780,000 fatalities per year.

Hepatitis B's global effects extend beyond its effects on health. It also puts a heavy financial strain on societies. The expenses incurred by healthcare providers, pharmaceutical companies, and employees who miss work due to illness are significant. Furthermore, because the disease can lead to societal stigma and prejudice against those who are affected, the effects on families and communities cannot be understated. Thankfully, there have been major developments in hepatitis B prevention and treatment. The prevalence of new infections has been successfully decreased by vaccination campaigns, particularly in young children and newborns. Antiviral drugs can also be used to treat the disease's symptoms and halt its progression. Ensuring that prevention, diagnostic, and treatment services are accessible to all people still presents difficulties. Many low- and middle-income nations still face challenges related to scarce resources and insufficient healthcare facilities.

This makes it more difficult to stop the spread of hepatitis B and treat individuals who need it quickly.

One of the primary reasons for these challenges is the limited funding available for healthcare in these nations. Often, a significant portion of their budget is allocated to other pressing needs such as infrastructure, education, and poverty alleviation. This results in inadequate investment in healthcare infrastructure, including hospitals, clinics, and laboratories, which are crucial for diagnosing and treating hepatitis B. Additionally, the scarcity of resources, such as medical equipment, diagnostic tools, and medications, further exacerbates the problem. Hepatitis B requires regular monitoring, prompt diagnosis, and access to antiviral medications, but these resources may be limited or unavailable in many low- and middle-income nations.

This lack of resources hinders the ability to provide timely and effective treatment to individuals with hepatitis B.

Moreover, there may be a shortage of healthcare professionals, including doctors, nurses, and laboratory technicians. This shortage can be attributed to factors like brain drain, where skilled healthcare professionals migrate to developed nations for better opportunities, leaving a void in their home countries. The lack of trained healthcare professionals limits the capacity to diagnose and treat hepatitis B cases promptly and adequately. Furthermore, the overall healthcare infrastructure and delivery systems in these nations may be underdeveloped or inefficient.

CHAPTER TWO

2.1 Biology and Transmission of Hepatitis B

A viral infection called hepatitis B damages the liver, causing inflammation and possibly long-term health issues. In order to stop the spread of hepatitis B and control its effects on people and communities, it is essential to comprehend its biology and mode of transmission. *We will examine the biology of the hepatitis B virus (HBV) and its mode of transmission in this article.*

2.2 Biology of Hepatitis B

The Hepadnaviridae family of viruses includes the tiny, partly double-stranded DNA virus that causes hepatitis B. It mainly targets hepatocytes, or liver cells, and is special in that it may incorporate its genetic material into the DNA of the host. This integration process can lead to persistent infection and impede the immune system's ability to fully eliminate the virus. The hepatitis B virus is composed of an outer envelope (HBsAg), an inner core (HBcAg) that contains the viral DNA, and reverse transcriptase, an enzyme that facilitates the virus's replication inside the host cell. Reverse transcription is the process by which viral DNA is changed from RNA to DNA again, enabling the creation of new viral particles.

2.3 Transmission of Hepatitis B

Hepatitis B can be transmitted through various means, including: **Blood contact**: Touching contaminated blood is the most typical way that the infection is spread. This can happen via exchanging tainted needles or other drug-related items, getting tainted blood transfusions, or being in direct contact with someone else's blood, such as through open wounds or cuts. When the blood of an infected person comes into contact with an open area on another person's body, there is a risk of transmission of infections, such as hepatitis B, hepatitis C, or HIV. It is important to take precautions and practice good hygiene to prevent the spread of these infections. This includes using clean and sterile equipment for medical procedures, avoiding sharing needles or drug paraphernalia, and practicing safe sexual behaviors. If you suspect that you have had contact with contaminated blood, it is important to seek medical advice and get tested for any potential infections.

2.4 Structure and Replication of the Hepatitis B Virus (HBV)

With millions of cases worldwide, it is a serious global health issue. Combating the virus and creating efficient treatment plans require an understanding of the structure and replication of HBV.

Structure of HBV: The HBV is a small, enveloped virus belonging to the family Hepadnaviridae. It has a unique structure that consists of several components:

1. Viral envelope: A lipid bilayer that is produced from the host cell membrane envelops the HBV. Viral proteins, including the surface antigen (HBsAg), which is involved in viral attachment and immunological detection, are present in this envelope.

2. Core structure: The viral DNA is contained within the envelope by a protein shell known as the core structure. The spherical structure of the core is formed by the self-assembly of core proteins (HBcAg).

3. Viral genome: The 3.2 kilobases that make up the HBV genome are circular DNA molecules that are partially double-stranded. The four overlapping open reading frames (ORFs) that make up this sequence encode different viral

proteins, such as the X, surface, polymerase, and core proteins.

Replication of HBV: Understanding the HBV replication mechanism is essential for formulating efficacious treatment plans and creating prophylactic interventions. *We shall examine the essential processes in HBV replication in this post.*

1. Entry into the host cell: Hepatocytes are the main target cells in the liver, where HBV enters. The virus enters the cell by attaching itself to particular cellular receptors on the surface of the hepatocyte.

2. Uncoating: HBV removes its outer membrane and releases its viral DNA into the cytoplasm of the host cell once it has entered the cell. Covalently closed circular DNA (cccDNA), a

partially double-stranded circular genome, is a type of viral DNA.

3. Transcription and translation: The transcription machinery of the host cell uses the cccDNA as a template to create viral RNA molecules. Viral proteins, such as the core antigen (HBcAg), surface antigen (HBsAg), and other enzymes needed for replication, are created by translating these RNA molecules.

4. Nucleocapsid assembly: A nucleocapsid, made up of the newly generated viral RNA and the core antigen, is formed. In addition to acting as a reverse transcription template, this nucleocapsid shields the viral DNA.

5. Reverse transcription: Reverse transcription is a crucial step in the replication process of the hepatitis B virus (HBV). During reverse

transcription, the viral RNA acts as a template for the synthesis of viral DNA. This process is facilitated by an enzyme called reverse transcriptase, which is carried by the HBV.

The reverse transcription process can be summarized as follows:

1. The HBV viral RNA enters the host cell and is transported to the cytoplasm.

2. Inside the cytoplasm, the viral RNA serves as a template for the reverse transcriptase enzyme.

3. Reverse transcriptase synthesizes a complementary DNA strand (cDNA) using the viral RNA as a template.

4. The cDNA synthesis occurs in a stepwise manner, starting from the 5' end of the viral RNA.

5. As the cDNA synthesis progresses, the viral RNA is

degraded by the RNase H activity of reverse transcriptase.

6. Once the full-length cDNA is synthesized, it forms a complete double-stranded DNA molecule.

7. The double-stranded DNA then enters the nucleus of the host cell and integrates into the host genome, forming a covalently closed circular DNA (cccDNA) molecule.

8. The cccDNA serves as a template for the synthesis of viral mRNA, which is then translated into viral proteins and used for the production of new viral particles.

Reverse transcription is a unique characteristic of HBV and some other retroviruses, where the viral RNA is converted into DNA before integration into the host cell's genome. This process is facilitated by an enzyme called reverse transcriptase, which is found in the viral particle. Reverse transcription is a crucial step in the life cycle of retroviruses like the hepatitis B virus (HBV) and the human immunodeficiency virus (HIV). These viruses have an RNA genome, but they need to convert their genetic material into DNA to effectively replicate and persist in the host cell.

When the virus enters the host cell, the reverse transcriptase enzyme synthesizes complementary DNA (cDNA) from the viral RNA template. This cDNA is then integrated into the host cell's genome, becoming a permanent part of the cell's genetic material. This integration allows the virus to exploit the host cell's machinery to produce new viral particles. The reverse transcription process has several implications for the persistence and treatment of HBV infection. Since the viral DNA becomes a part of the host cell's genome, it can remain in the body for a long time, even after the initial infection has resolved. This is why HBV infections can sometimes become chronic and persist for years, leading to liver damage and other complications.

Furthermore, the reverse transcription process presents a challenge in antiviral therapy development. Most antiviral drugs target viral enzymes or processes specific to the virus, but reverse transcriptase is also involved in the normal functioning of the host cell. Developing drugs that selectively inhibit viral reverse transcriptase without harming host cell enzymes is a complex task.

2.5 Modes of Transmission

In the realm of medicine, knowing how illnesses spread is essential to putting preventative measures in place and halting the spread of infections. Different diseases can spread in different ways, and understanding these ways can assist both individuals and medical professionals in taking the appropriate preventative measures. The following are some typical means of transmission:

1. Direct Contact: Direct contact with an infected individual or their body fluids can result in the spread of many infectious diseases. This covers physical contact such as kissing, hugging, and even sneezing and coughing up droplets. HIV and other sexually transmitted viruses, as well as the common cold, are

examples of diseases that can be spread via direct contact.

2. Indirect Contact: When a person comes into contact with a contaminated surface or object, this is known as indirect contact. Because the germs are able to thrive on these surfaces, when someone touches their lips or face, the infection can spread. Indirect contact can result in the transmission of diseases such as norovirus, the flu, and certain forms of food poisoning.

3. Airborne Transmission: A few infectious diseases have the ability to transmit through minuscule particles or droplet nuclei that hang out in the atmosphere for extended periods of time. People who are close to an infected person or who are in enclosed settings with inadequate ventilation may inhale these infections. Airborne transmission is the means by which

respiratory infections such as COVID-19 and tuberculosis are transmitted.

4. Vector-Borne Transmission: Certainly! Vector-borne transmission refers to the process by which certain diseases are transmitted to humans or animals through the bites of infected arthropods, such as fleas, ticks, mosquitoes, and other insects. These vectors act as carriers or conduits for the pathogens that cause various diseases. However, it's important to note that hepatitis B is not primarily transmitted through vector-borne means. While mosquitoes are known to transmit other diseases like malaria, dengue fever, or the Zika virus, they are not known to be vectors for hepatitis B.

5. Bloodborne transmission: Coming into contact with contaminated blood can spread hepatitis B. Blood

transfusions, sharing needles or other drug paraphernalia, and unintentional needlestick injuries can all lead to this. Healthcare professionals and anyone else who might come into contact with blood should take the appropriate safety measures to stop the spread of the infection.

6. Sexual contact with an infected person can result in the transfer of hepatitis B. Unprotected sexual activity can carry a risk of transmission, including oral, anal, and vaginal sex. To lower the risk of infection, barrier techniques like condoms are crucial.

7. Mother-to-child transmission: During childbirth, an infected mother may transmit hepatitis B to her unborn child. If the newborn receives the hepatitis B vaccine and immunoglobulin within 12 hours of birth, the risk of transmission can be greatly decreased.

8. Sharing personal objects: Hepatitis B can be spread by sharing personal goods, including razors, toothbrushes, and anything that might come into contact with blood. Sharing such products should be avoided, particularly if you live with someone who is infected or don't know if they are positive for hepatitis B.

9. Occupational exposure: healthcare workers or individuals working in environments. For those who work in healthcare settings or in jobs involving blood or body fluids, occupational exposure to hepatitis B is a serious risk. If left untreated, the viral infection known as hepatitis B can cause cirrhosis, liver cancer, or chronic liver disease. Due to their frequent contact with patients' bodily fluids, healthcare workers including doctors, nurses, laboratory technicians, and

emergency personnel—are more likely to contract hepatitis B at work. Blood sample handling laboratory workers, tattoo artists, dentists, and inmates are among the other professions that could be in danger.

It is imperative to prevent occupational exposure to hepatitis B, and there are several ways to do this. Vaccination is the best defense against the spread of hepatitis B. The hepatitis B vaccination series, which consists of three doses administered over a six-month period, should be administered to all healthcare workers and persons who are at risk. Vaccination lowers the chance of infection and offers long-term protection against the virus. Healthcare personnel should adhere to stringent infection control procedures in addition to vaccinations to reduce the chance of exposure. Wearing personal protective equipment (PPE) such as gowns, gloves, masks, and eye protection is part of this, especially while working with patients or doing operations that might come into contact with body fluids like blood. To stop the virus from spreading, practice good hand hygiene, which includes often washing your hands with soap and water or using hand sanitizers with alcohol in them. If a person contracts hepatitis B at work, they should take quick action.

2.6 Risk Factors for Hepatitis B Transmission

Understanding Prevention Strategies: In order to put effective preventative measures into practice, it is essential to comprehend the risk factors for hepatitis B transmission. In this piece, we'll examine the main risk factors for the development of hepatitis B and talk about ways to stop the infection from spreading.

1. Unprotected Sexual Contact: Having intercourse without protection greatly raises the risk of infection, particularly when doing so with several partners or people who are hepatitis B positive. The virus can easily spread during sexual activity because it can be found in seminal and vaginal fluids.

2. Prevention: The risk of hepatitis B transmission can be significantly decreased by practicing safe sex and using barrier techniques like condoms. It is also advised that both partners receive vaccinations.

3. Sharing Needles or Syringes: Using injection drugs increases the chance of contracting hepatitis B. The

virus can enter the bloodstream through direct blood exchange caused by sharing syringes or needles with infected people.

4. Prevention: To reduce the risk, promote the use of sterile needles and syringes and ask for aid from harm reduction organizations. It's also critical to provide hepatitis B vaccines to drug injectors.

5. Perinatal Transmission: During birth, pregnant women who have a hepatitis B infection might pass the virus to their unborn child.

CHAPTER THREE

3.1 Epidemiology and Prevalence of Hepatitis B

The hepatitis B virus (HBV) is the source of hepatitis B, a viral infection that is a serious global public health concern. For successful prevention, diagnosis, and treatment plans, it is essential to comprehend the epidemiology and prevalence of this illness. The purpose of this is to shed light on the prevalence rates, risk factors, and transmission of hepatitis B, as well as its global effects.

Transmission: The main way that hepatitis B is spread is by contact with contaminated blood or bodily fluids, which can happen during unprotected sexual contact, sharing of needles, or delivery when an infected mother gives birth to her child. Additionally, using contaminated medical equipment or intimate domestic contact can spread it.

Global Prevalence: The prevalence of hepatitis B varies around the world and is endemic in many areas. In 2019, the World Health Organization (WHO) estimated that 257 million people worldwide were chronically infected with hepatitis B. Up to 5% of adults in the Western Pacific and sub-Saharan Africa regions have chronic infections, which correspond to the greatest prevalence rates.

Risk Factors: Hepatitis B is more likely to infect certain populations. These include those who inject drugs, have unprotected sex, work in healthcare facilities where blood and bodily fluids are handled, and have babies delivered to infected moms. Furthermore, those who reside in places with inadequate sanitation and restricted access to healthcare facilities are more vulnerable to the HBV.

3.2 Global Burden of Hepatitis B

Hepatitis B's global burden is a serious public health concern that impacts millions of individuals globally. The virus that causes hepatitis B mainly targets the liver, inflaming it and raising the risk of life-threatening side effects such as liver cirrhosis and liver cancer. To effectively prevent, diagnose, and treat hepatitis B, it is imperative to comprehend the disease's worldwide prevalence. In 2019, the World Health Organization (WHO) estimated that 257 million people worldwide were chronically infected with hepatitis B. Given that persistent infections can have long-term health effects and increase the death rate associated with liver illnesses, this represents a substantial worldwide burden. About 900,000 deaths are attributed to hepatitis B each year, most of which are caused by complications, including cirrhosis and liver cancer. Worldwide, the prevalence of hepatitis B is not uniform. East Asia and sub-Saharan Africa have the highest prevalence rates, with up to 10% of the population potentially living with a chronic infection. These areas are regarded as endemic for hepatitis B, which indicates that the virus is pervasive and can be passed from mother to child or by contact with contaminated bodily fluids like blood.

The four main pillars of the global hepatitis B epidemic strategy are prevention, immunization, screening, and treatment. The best defense against hepatitis B infection is vaccination, which is advised for high-risk individuals and all newborns. In order to enable early intervention and treatment, screening programs assist in identifying those who are affected.

3.3 Regional Variations in Hepatitis B Prevalence

The viral infection known as hepatitis B damages the liver and varies greatly in frequency among different geographical areas of the world.

Effective prevention and control efforts, as well as the provision of appropriate healthcare services to afflicted communities, depend on an understanding of these geographical variations. We'll look at a few of the main causes of the regional differences in the frequency of hepatitis B here.

Endemic vs. Non-Endemic Regions: The high transmission rates and early onset of infection in many parts of Asia and Africa make hepatitis B an endemic disease. Compared to non-endemic areas like North America and Western Europe, these locations often have a greater frequency of chronic hepatitis B infection.

Modes of Transmission: Hepatitis B can spread by a number of methods, such as exposure to contaminated blood, sharing of syringes or needles, unprotected sexual contact, and transmission from an infected mother to her unborn child. The prevalence of hepatitis B can be significantly influenced by the routes of transmission that are common in a certain area.

Immunization Coverage: One of the most important factors in lowering the incidence of the disease is the accessibility and availability of hepatitis B immunization programs. Hepatitis B infection rates are often lower in areas with high vaccination rates, particularly among young children. This is especially true in nations where routine childhood immunization schedules incorporate the hepatitis B vaccine into national immunization programs.

3.4 High-Risk Populations and Vulnerable Groups Living with Hepatitis B

The disease is thought to be more likely to affect or weaken specific populations. We will examine the disadvantaged and high-risk populations affected by hepatitis B, outlining the particular difficulties they encounter and the significance of focused interventions and support.

Injecting Drug Users: The risk of acquiring hepatitis B is considerably higher for those who use injectable drugs. The virus can spread through sharing contaminated needles or drug paraphernalia. The main focus of public health activities should be harm reduction tactics, such as education, testing, immunization, and treatment service accessibility, as well as needle exchange programs.

Men who have Sex with Men (MSM): In comparison to the general population, MSM have a greater prevalence of hepatitis B. Unprotected sexual activity, having several partners, and having additional STDs are risk factors. To lower the transmission rates among this susceptible population, targeted outreach initiatives that encourage safe sexual practices, frequent testing, and immunization are crucial.

Migrants and Refugees: There is a higher incidence of hepatitis B among migrants and refugees, among other particular healthcare issues. Lack of knowledge about treatment and preventative alternatives, cultural views, language obstacles, and restricted access to healthcare are some of the factors that raise risk. It is essential to have thorough screening, immunizations, and culturally competent support services.

CHAPTER FOUR

4.1 Clinical Manifestations of Hepatitis B

The liver is the main organ affected by the viral infection known as hepatitis B. The hepatitis B virus (HBV) is the cause, and it can present with a variety of clinical symptoms. Comprehending the clinical presentations of hepatitis B is crucial for prompt identification, handling, and averting consequences. The following are the main clinical signs and symptoms of hepatitis B:

4.2 Asymptomatic Infection

Asymptomatic infections are common in hepatitis B patients, particularly in the early phases of the illness. This kind of infection is known as asymptomatic. These people might still be virus carriers who can spread the infection to other people.

4.3 Acute Hepatitis

The term "acute" hepatitis B describes the first infection, which typically lasts anywhere from a few weeks to many months. Many infected individuals may not show any symptoms at all during this phase of the virus's life, but some may experience flu-like symptoms include lethargy, appetite loss, nausea, vomiting, jaundice (yellowing of the skin and eyes), light-colored feces, dark urine, stomach discomfort, and occasionally fever. Usually, these signs appear one to six months following viral exposure. Acute hepatitis B can occasionally develop into a chronic infection that lasts longer than six months. Serious side effects from chronic hepatitis B include liver failure, liver malignancy, and cirrhosis (liver scarring). Roughly 25% of people with chronic hepatitis B are predicted to experience these serious side effects.

4.4 Chronic Hepatitis

If the infection persists for longer than six months, it is referred to as chronic hepatitis B. Long-term liver damage, such as liver cirrhosis and hepatocellular carcinoma, can be brought on by persistent infection. Many people with chronic hepatitis B may not show any symptoms at first, but they may eventually encounter liver dysfunction-related problems.

4.5 Transmission

Transmission: Hepatitis B is primarily spread through contact with infected blood or other body fluids. It can also be spread through unprotected sexual activity, sharing needles or syringes, and from an infected mother to her baby during childbirth. 5. Symptoms: The symptoms of acute hepatitis B can vary and include fatigue, loss of appetite, nausea, vomiting, abdominal pain, dark urine, jaundice (yellowing of the skin and eyes), joint pain, and fatigue.

Symptoms: The symptoms of acute hepatitis B can vary and may include fatigue, loss of appetite, nausea, vomiting, abdominal pain, dark urine, jaundice (yellowing of the skin and eyes), and joint pain. However, some individuals may experience mild or even no symptoms.

Diagnosis: A blood test is usually performed to diagnose acute hepatitis B. This test looks for specific antibodies or antigens related to the virus (Check 5.1),

4.6 Understanding Chronic Hepatitis B: Causes, Symptoms, and Treatment Options

Chronic Hepatitis B is a serious liver infection caused by the Hepatitis B virus (HBV). It is a worldwide health concern, affecting millions of people and is a leading cause of liver disease, liver cancer, and liver failure. This ia aims to provide an overview of Chronic Hepatitis B, including its causes, symptoms, and available treatment options.

Causes of Chronic Hepatitis B

The hepatitis B virus is the main cause of chronic hepatitis B. Most often, HIV spreads through unprotected sexual contact, contact with contaminated blood, or childbirth from an infected mother to her child. Additionally, sharing infected toothbrushes, razors, or needles can spread the virus.

Chronic Hepatitis B Symptoms

Many people with chronic hepatitis B may not show any symptoms at all, especially in the early stages of the illness. However, if the infection worsens, a few typical signs and symptoms could appear, such as:

1. Weakness and exhaustion.

2. Appetite loss.

3. Throwing up and feeling queasy.

4. Pain in the abdomen.

5. Jaundice (eye and skin yellowing) 6. Dark urine.

7. Sore joints.

8. Extended fever.

9. Easy bleeding or bruises

It is important to note that symptoms can vary from person to person, and some individuals may remain asymptomatic for years while still carrying the virus.

Hepatitis B Related Complications

While many individuals with Hepatitis B experience mild symptoms or even no symptoms at all, some may develop complications that can have a significant impact on their health. *Here are some of the complications associated with Hepatitis B:*

1. Hepatitis B is a risk factor for liver cirrhosis, a disorder marked by the scarring of the liver's tissue. The liver gets harder with time, which makes it harder for it to work correctly. Numerous consequences, including liver failure, portal hypertension (high blood pressure in the liver), and an elevated risk of liver cancer, can result from cirrhosis.

2. Liver Cancer: Hepatocellular carcinoma, another name for liver cancer, is considerably more likely to

occur in people who have a chronic Hepatitis B infection. Regular tests are crucial for people with chronic hepatitis B in order to identify any indications of liver cancer early on, when treatment choices are more successful.

3. Fulminant Hepatitis: Hepatitis B can occasionally result in fulminant hepatitis, a serious and potentially fatal illness. This happens when the liver's ability to function is abruptly and drastically lost. If left untreated, fulminant hepatitis can necessitate a liver transplant.

4. Kidney issues: Membranous glomerulonephritis and membranoproliferative glomerulonephritis are two kidney issues that have been linked to hepatitis B. There is inflammation associated with certain illnesses.

CHAPTER FIVE

5.1 Diagnosis and Monitoring of Hepatitis B

Diagnosis and monitoring of hepatitis B play a crucial role in effectively managing the disease and preventing its complications. Hepatitis B is a viral infection that affects the liver and can lead to chronic liver disease, liver failure, or liver cancer if left untreated. Early detection and monitoring of the infection are essential for timely intervention and appropriate medical management. *Here are some important aspects of the diagnosis and monitoring of Hepatitis B:*

Screening: The first step in diagnosis is to identify individuals who may be at risk of Hepatitis B. This includes individuals with a history of exposure to the virus, such as those born to infected mothers, individuals with a history of unprotected sexual activity, healthcare workers, and intravenous drug users. Screening tests involve the detection of specific hepatitis B surface antigens and antibodies in the blood.

Confirmation: Additional testing is done to confirm the diagnosis if the screening test yields positive results. This entails measuring the hepatitis B core antigen, liver function tests, and viral DNA levels. The degree of viral replication and the infection's stage (acute or chronic) can both be ascertained with confirmation.

Liver Function Tests: These tests evaluate the liver's general health and can assist in estimating the extent of liver damage brought on by the infection. These tests quantify a range of blood components, including proteins, enzymes, and chemicals, that are suggestive of liver function.

Serological markers: such as hepatitis B surface antigen, are substances present in the blood that can indicate the presence of a particular infection or disease. These markers are typically proteins or other molecules produced by the body in response to an infection or as a result of an autoimmune disorder. In the case of hepatitis B, the presence of the hepatitis B surface antigen (HBsAg) in a person's blood indicates that they are currently infected with the hepatitis B virus. This marker is commonly tested for in screenings for hepatitis B and is used to diagnose acute or chronic hepatitis B infections.

Serological markers play a crucial role in diagnosing and monitoring various diseases and infections. They help healthcare professionals determine the specific disease or condition a patient may have and track their progress during treatment. This information is essential for making informed decisions about treatment options and managing patient care effectively.

5.2 Screening and Diagnostic Tests for Hepatitis B

If left untreated, hepatitis B, a viral illness that affects the liver, can cause major health problems. Tests for screening and diagnosis are essential for determining whether a person has the hepatitis B virus

(HBV). These tests assist medical professionals in diagnosing the infection and choosing the best course of action for management and treatment. *Here are some details regarding hepatitis B screening and diagnosis procedures:*

1. Hepatitis B Surface Antigen (HBsAg) Test:

The most used test for hepatitis B screening is this one. It determines whether the blood contains HBV surface antigen. An active HBV infection is indicated by a positive HBsAg test result.

2. Hepatitis B Core Antibody (anti-HBc) Test:

This test detects the presence of antibodies against the core antigen of the Hepatitis B virus. It helps determine if a person has ever been infected with HBV, even if they have cleared the infection or are currently infected.

3. **Hepatitis B Surface Antibody (anti-HBs) Test**: This test measures the level of antibodies against the HBV surface antigen. It is commonly used to determine if a person has immunity to hepatitis B, either through vaccination or past infection.

4. **Hepatitis B Antigen (HBeAg) Test**: This test detects the presence of HBeAg, which is a marker for active viral replication. It helps determine if a person with Hepatitis B is highly infectious.

5. The Hepatitis B DNA Test, also known as PCR (Polymerase Chain Reaction), is a diagnostic test used to detect and measure the presence of Hepatitis B virus (HBV) in a person's blood. PCR is a highly sensitive and specific technique that amplifies the viral DNA in a blood sample, making it easier to detect even small

amounts of the virus. This test can accurately determine the viral load (the amount of virus present in the blood) and assess the severity of the infection. *The hepatitis B DNA test is commonly used to:*

Diagnose Hepatitis B infection: It can detect the presence of HBV in individuals who are suspected of being infected. It is especially useful in cases where other tests, such as antibody tests, may not provide definitive results.

Monitor disease progression: The test can measure the level of viral replication in chronically infected individuals over time. It helps healthcare providers understand if the infection is getting better or worse and guides treatment decisions.

Evaluate treatment efficacy: PCR testing is used to assess the effectiveness of antiviral therapies in suppressing HBV replication. By monitoring the viral load, doctors can determine if the treatment is working or if adjustments are needed. It is important to note that the hepatitis B DNA test should be performed by a qualified healthcare professional in a laboratory setting. to ensure that the individual executing the test possesses the necessary knowledge and skills to handle and interpret the results accurately. This is crucial to ensuring the reliability and validity of the test outcomes. Moreover, conducting the hepatitis B DNA test in a laboratory setting ensures that the test is performed using standardized procedures and equipment. This minimizes the chances of errors or contamination that could potentially affect the accuracy of the results.

The results of the hepatitis B DNA test should be considered in conjunction with other clinical information. This means that the test results should be interpreted by a healthcare professional who can take into account the individual's medical history, symptoms, and other relevant factors to make an accurate diagnosis and provide appropriate treatment recommendations. Overall, the emphasis on qualified professionals, laboratory settings, and the integration of test results with other clinical information underscores the importance of accurate testing and diagnosis when it comes to hepatitis B.

Interpretation of Hepatitis B Test Results

Hepatitis B is a viral infection that primarily affects the liver. It is important to interpret the results of hepatitis B tests accurately to assess the infection status and determine appropriate management strategies. Here is a guide to interpreting Hepatitis B test results:

Hepatitis B Surface Antigen (HBsAg):

Positive result: A positive HBsAg indicates an active Hepatitis B infection. Further tests may be required to assess the stage of the infection and determine the need for treatment.

Negative result: A negative HBsAg suggests the absence of a current Hepatitis B infection. However, it is vital to consider other markers to confirm the infection status, especially in individuals with a known history of exposure.

Hepatitis B Surface Antibody (anti-HBs)

Positive result: A positive anti-HBs antibody indicates that the individual has developed immunity to Hepatitis B either through a natural infection or vaccination.

Negative result: A negative anti-HBs suggests the absence of protective antibodies against Hepatitis B. This may indicate a need for vaccination or further evaluation, especially in high-risk individuals.

Hepatitis B Core Antibody (anti-HBc)

IgM anti-HBc: A positive result for IgM anti-HBc suggests an acute or recent Hepatitis B infection. IgG anti-HBc refers to immunoglobulin G antibodies against the hepatitis B core antigen (HBcAg). When a test result shows a positive result for IgG anti-HBc, it indicates that the person has been exposed to the hepatitis B virus (HBV) in the past. The presence of IgG anti-HBc antibodies means that the person has either had a previous HBV infection that has resolved or has received a hepatitis B vaccine. These antibodies typically remain in the body for a long time, even after the infection has cleared or the vaccination has been administered.

It is important to note that a positive IgG anti-HBc result does not indicate a current or active infection. To determine the current status of hepatitis B infection, additional tests such as HBsAg (hepatitis B surface antigen) and anti-HBs (antibodies against hepatitis B surface antigen) may be required. *If you have further questions or concerns about hepatitis B testing, it is best to consult with a healthcare professional or a specialist in infectious diseases.*

5.3 Monitoring Hepatitis B Infection and Disease Progression

A hepatitis B infection is a viral infection that primarily affects the liver. It can lead to both acute and chronic liver disease, with potential long-term consequences such as cirrhosis, liver failure, and hepatocellular carcinoma. Monitoring the progression of hepatitis B infection is crucial for effective disease management and the prevention of complications.

Regular medical check-ups: Individuals diagnosed with hepatitis B should undergo regular medical check-ups to monitor the progress of the infection. This includes physical examinations, blood tests, and imaging studies to assess liver health and functioning.

Liver Function Tests: A blood test called a liver function test (LFT) assesses the liver's capacity to carry out its duties. LFTs measure a range of blood components, including proteins, enzymes, and chemicals, that signify inflammation or injury to the liver. These examinations aid in determining the extent of hepatitis B infection and tracking the disease's advancement over time.

Hepatitis B Viral Load Testing: This test quantifies the bloodstream's concentration of the hepatitis B virus (HBV). It aids in estimating the degree of viral replication and evaluating the efficacy of antiviral treatment. It is necessary to monitor the HBV viral load in order to modify treatment regimens and assess the effectiveness of antiviral drugs.

Hepatitis B Antigen (HBeAg) and Hepatitis B Surface Antigen (HBsAg) Testing: HBeAg and HBsAg are important markers used to monitor hepatitis B infection.

CHAPTER SIX

6.1 Treatment Options for Hepatitis B: Managing and Controlling the Infection

Hepatitis B is a viral infection that affects the liver, caused by the hepatitis B virus (HBV). It can lead to both acute and chronic liver disease, ranging from mild illness to severe complications. Treatment for hepatitis B aims to control the infection, prevent liver damage, and reduce the risk of developing long-term complications. In this article, we will explore the various treatment options available for managing and treating hepatitis B.

Antiviral Drugs: The mainstay of treatment for hepatitis B is antiviral drugs. These drugs suppress the infection by lessening the hepatitis B virus's ability to replicate within the body. Antiviral medications for hepatitis B are frequently used and include:

a) Tenofovir alafenamide (TAF) and tenofovir disoproxil fumarate (TDF): These medications are very good at preventing viral replication and lowering hepatic inflammation. For the treatment of chronic hepatitis B, they are regarded as first-line alternatives.

b) Another strong antiviral medication used to treat chronic hepatitis B is entecavir. It aids in the management of the infection by preventing viral multiplication.

c) Interferons: Interferons are a type of immunotherapy used to treat various viral infections, including the hepatitis B virus (HBV). Interferons are proteins naturally produced by the immune system in response to viral infections. They have antiviral properties and help stimulate the body's immune response. In the case of hepatitis B, interferons can be administered to help strengthen the body's defenses against the virus. Interferons work by activating certain immune cells, such as natural killer cells and T-cells, which play a crucial role in fighting off viral infections. By stimulating the immune system, interferons can help slow down the replication of the hepatitis B virus, reduce liver inflammation, and prevent further liver damage. They can also help increase the body's production of antibodies that specifically target the hepatitis B virus.

Note that interferon therapy is not suitable for everyone and can have side effects. Common side effects include flu-like symptoms, fatigue, depression, and gastrointestinal issues. This treatment approach is typically considered for individuals with chronic hepatitis B who meet specific criteria, such as having certain liver function tests and a certain level of hepatitis B viral load.

c) Interferons: An immunotherapy treatment known as interferons helps strengthen the body's defenses against the hepatitis B virus. They can be used for both acute and chronic infections, and they are usually given as injections.

6.2 Regular Monitoring and

Screening

Chronic hepatitis B (CHB) is a viral infection that affects the liver, causing inflammation and potentially leading to severe complications such as liver cirrhosis and hepatocellular carcinoma. Over the years, significant advancements have been made in the development of antiviral therapies, revolutionizing the treatment landscape for CHB patients. In this article, we will explore the different antiviral therapies available for managing chronic hepatitis B and the impact they have on patients' lives.

Nucleoside Analogs (NAs): Nucleotide analogs like entecavir and tenofovir disoproxil fumarate are considered first-line therapies for CHB.

These medications work by inhibiting the replication of the hepatitis B virus (HBV) in the body, thus reducing viral load and liver inflammation. NAs are highly effective and can suppress the virus to undetectable levels, improving liver function and reducing the risk of disease progression.

Interferon-Based Therapies: Interferon-based therapies, such as pegylated interferon-alpha, stimulate the body's immune response against HBV. These therapies have both antiviral and immunomodulatory properties, making them beneficial for select CHB patients. Interferon-based therapies are usually administered over a fixed period, and their treatment outcomes may vary from patient to patient.

6.3 Antiviral Therapies for Chronic Hepatitis B: Promising Advances in Treatment

A global health concern that affects millions of individuals globally is chronic hepatitis B (CHB). The Hepatitis B virus (HBV) is the origin of this dangerous liver infection, which can have long-term consequences such as liver cirrhosis, liver failure, and hepatocellular cancer. Although there is still no known cure for CHB, great strides have been made in the creation of antiviral medications that can successfully control the illness and enhance patient outcomes. We shall examine the most recent developments in antiviral treatments for chronic Hepatitis B in this post.

Nucleos(t)ide Analogs (NAs): The foundation of the antiviral therapy for CHB is NAs. They function by preventing the HBV DNA from replicating, lowering the viral load, and delaying the onset of liver damage. Tenofovir and entecavir are two often used NAs that have demonstrated good effectiveness in reducing viral replication and enhancing liver function. It has been demonstrated that long-term NA therapy lowers the risk of hepatocellular cancer, liver cirrhosis, and the requirement for liver transplantation.

Pegylated Interferon-alpha (PEG-IFNα): In order to help the body fight off an HBV infection, PEG-IFNα is an immune modulator. It functions by preventing the spread of the virus and encouraging the removal of infected people.

6.4 Management of Acute Hepatitis

The hallmark of acute hepatitis is the abrupt onset of liver inflammation, which is typically brought on by viral infections such as hepatitis A, B, C, D, or E. In order to avoid complications and encourage recovery, acute hepatitis must be treated promptly and appropriately. The goal of this article is to present a thorough management strategy for acute hepatitis, covering diagnosis, therapy, and supportive care.

Diagnosis: Clinical evaluation: To identify the cause and severity of acute hepatitis, a complete medical history, physical examination, and assessment of risk factors are crucial.

Laboratory studies: Specific hepatitis markers, viral serology, and blood tests to evaluate liver function all help to confirm the diagnosis and pinpoint the virus causing it.

Treatment

Supportive care: Adequate rest, proper nutrition, and hydration are vital for patients with acute hepatitis. Alcohol and hepatotoxic medications should be avoided.

Antiviral therapy: Depending on the specific hepatitis virus, antiviral medications may be prescribed to suppress viral replication and reduce liver inflammation. The choice of antiviral therapy depends on the type and severity of the infection.

Immune modulators: In some cases, immune-modulating medications may be used to manage severe or fulminant hepatitis, aiming to reduce immune-mediated liver injury.

6.5 Understanding the Link Between Hepatitis B and Liver Cancer

Liver cancer, or hepatocellular carcinoma (HCC), is a serious condition that affects millions of people worldwide. While there are various risk factors associated with liver cancer, one of the leading causes is chronic infection with the hepatitis B virus (HBV). In this article, we will explore the connection between HBV and liver cancer, the risk factors, preventive measures, and available treatment options. Chronic HBV infection significantly increases the risk of developing liver cancer. HBV is responsible for causing liver inflammation, cell damage, and the formation of cancerous cells over time. It is estimated that around 20–30% of individuals chronically infected with HBV will eventually develop liver cancer.

Risk Factors: Individuals with chronic HBV infection are at a higher risk of developing liver cancer compared to those without the infection. Other factors that can increase the risk include alcohol consumption, smoking, obesity, exposure to aflatoxins (a type of toxin produced by mold), and co-infection with the hepatitis C virus (HCV).

Preventive Measures:

The hepatitis B vaccine is highly effective in preventing HBV infection and subsequently reducing the risk of liver cancer. It is recommended for all individuals, especially those at higher risk.

6.6 Understanding Liver Cancer in Hepatitis B Patients: Causes

Liver cancer, also known as hepatocellular carcinoma (HCC), is a serious condition that can develop in individuals with a chronic hepatitis B infection. Hepatitis B is a viral infection that primarily affects the liver, and when left untreated, it can lead to liver damage and potentially cancerous growths. In this article, we will delve into the causes, symptoms, and treatment options for liver cancer in hepatitis B patients.

Causes: Chronic hepatitis B infection is the primary cause of liver cancer in individuals worldwide. The hepatitis B virus (HBV) attacks liver cells, causing inflammation and scarring. Over time, this chronic inflammation can lead to the development of cancerous cells in the liver.

The risk of liver cancer increases in patients who have been infected with hepatitis B for a long time, especially if they have not received proper medical management. Other factors, such as family history of liver cancer, co-infection with hepatitis C or HIV, alcohol abuse, and exposure to certain toxins, can further increase the risk.

Symptoms: Liver cancer often presents with vague symptoms, especially in the early stages. Some common symptoms include:

1. unexplained weight loss

2. Fatigue and weakness

3. Abdominal pain or discomfort

4. loss of appetite

5. Jaundice (yellowing of the skin and eyes)

6. swelling in the abdomen or legs.

6.7 Hepatitis B Vaccination: Protecting Against a Silent Threat

The hepatitis B virus (HBV) is the source of hepatitis B, a potentially dangerous liver infection. It might be a short-lived, moderate ailment that goes away in a few weeks or a chronic one that can cause liver damage, cirrhosis, or even liver cancer. The good news is that there is a vaccine that can guard against this quiet, possibly fatal infection, and it is safe and effective.

1. Knowledge about Hepatitis B: Blood or other bodily fluids from an infected individual can spread the virus. It can be transferred from an infected mother to her

newborn during childbirth, through sharing needles or other drug paraphernalia, or through unprotected sexual contact. Since many HBV patients may not exhibit any symptoms, early detection and prevention are essential.

2. The Benefits of Vaccination: The best defense against hepatitis B is vaccination. The vaccination triggers the production of antiviral antibodies by the body's immune system. Getting vaccinated helps prevent the virus from spreading throughout the community, in addition to protecting you.

3. Who needs vaccination?

Infants: Two more doses of the hepatitis B vaccine should be administered during infancy after the first dose, which should be administered soon after delivery.

Youngsters and Teens: If a person was not vaccinated as an infant, they should have the shot in childhood or adolescence.

Risky Adults: People who are more vulnerable include those who work in healthcare and those who have several sexual partners.

Safe Sex Practices for Hepatitis B Prevention: Sexual contact is one of the many ways that hepatitis B, a virus that damages the liver, can be spread. It's essential to use safe sexual practices to keep Hepatitis B from spreading and to safeguard both you and your partner. We'll talk about several crucial safe sex behaviors in this article that can lower the chance of spreading Hepatitis B.

1. Consistent and Correct Condom Use: One of the best strategies to stop the spread of Hepatitis B during

sexual activity is to use condoms correctly and consistently. Condoms made of latex or polyurethane offer great protection against the spread of bodily fluids that could harbor the Hepatitis B virus.

2. Vaccination: Getting vaccinated is crucial to avoiding contracting Hepatitis B. Ensure that you and your companion have received the Hepatitis B vaccination. The vaccination is widely accessible, safe, and efficient. It reduces the chance of virus transmission through sexual contact and offers long-term protection against it.

3. Communication and Disclosure: Having open and sincere conversations about sex with your partner is essential to safe sex practices. Talk to your partner about any possible concerns and your status regarding hepatitis B. Take the appropriate safety measures to

prevent sharing the virus with your partner if you or they are positive for Hepatitis B. This is especially important when engaging in unprotected sexual activity.

When it comes to halting the spread of Hepatitis B, needle and syringe safety is critical. The liver is the main organ affected by the highly contagious viral infection known as hepatitis B. Sharing contaminated needles or syringes is one of the major ways that HIV spreads. HIV can also be transmitted by contact with infected blood or other bodily fluids. *Several safety precautions should be taken in order to stop the spread of Hepatitis B via the use of needles and syringes:*

1. Always use sterile, fresh needles and syringes. Make sure that every injection is administered with brand-new needles and syringes. Needles should not be

shared or reused since this greatly raises the risk of hepatitis B transmission.

2. Correct disposal: Needles and syringes should be disposed of properly in a container that can withstand punctures after use. This aids in preventing unintentional needlestick injuries that may transmit Hepatitis B.

3. Universal precautions: When handling needles and syringes, healthcare personnel should follow universal precautions, which include donning gloves, masks, and other protective gear. Through these procedures, the danger of coming into contact with blood and other potentially infectious materials is reduced.

4. Safe injection techniques: It's critical to adhere to safe injection techniques when giving injections. This entails giving each patient their own needle and

syringe, refraining from recapping needles, and thoroughly cleaning the injection site before giving the medication.

5. Education and awareness: Hepatitis B education and awareness are essential for both controlling and preventing this viral infection. The hepatitis B virus (HBV) is the cause of hepatitis B, a dangerous liver illness. Contact with an infected person's blood or other bodily fluids can spread the infection.

When it comes to hepatitis B education and awareness, keep the following points in mind:

1. Comprehending the Illness: Disseminating knowledge about hepatitis B to the general public entails supplying details on the characteristics of the virus, its modes of transmission, and the possible

health ramifications. This includes describing the ways in which unprotected sexual contact, sharing syringes or needles, mother-to-child transmission during childbirth, and contact with contaminated bodily fluids or blood can all result in the transfer of HBV.

2. Preventive Measures: It's critical to spread knowledge about preventive measures. This includes pushing for the appropriate disposal of needles and syringes, urging people to get vaccinated against hepatitis B, and supporting the use of sterile equipment in healthcare settings.

3. Testing and Diagnosis: It's critical to inform people about the value of testing and prompt diagnosis. People should be informed about the advantages of early detection and the fact that screening tests for hepatitis B are readily available. This may result in

prompt medical attention and effective infection control.

4. Vaccine Campaigns: One important component of education and awareness is the promotion of the hepatitis B vaccine. urging people to be vaccinated, especially those who are at a higher risk, like healthcare professionals, newborns whose moms are infected, and those

6.8 Screening of Blood and Blood Products for Hepatitis B

If left untreated, hepatitis B, a viral illness that affects the liver, can cause serious health problems. Strict screening protocols are in place to guarantee the safety of recipients and stop the spread of Hepatitis B through blood transfusions and blood products. The hepatitis B virus (HBV) can be found in donated blood or blood products through a series of procedures in the screening process. The following are the main facets of the screening procedure:

1. Donor Questionnaire: Applicants for blood donations must answer a thorough series of questions about their health history, way of life, and possible exposure to hepatitis B. This makes it easier to identify those who could be more likely to carry the virus.

2. Laboratory Testing: To identify the presence of the Hepatitis B surface antigen (HBsAg), blood samples obtained from donors are subjected to extensive laboratory testing. The first and most accurate indicator of either an acute or chronic Hepatitis B

infection is HBsAg. Donated blood or blood products are disposed of if HBsAg is found.

3. Extra Testing: To further assess the existence of Hepatitis B, extra testing may occasionally be carried out. Hepatitis B surface antibody (anti-HBs) and hepatitis B core antibody (anti-HBc) measurements are among the tests that may be performed. The outcomes of these tests aid in establishing if the donor is immune due to vaccination, whether they have had an infection in the past or present, or both.

If left untreated, hepatitis B, a viral infection that affects the liver, can result in chronic liver disease. Fortunately, hepatitis B can be properly managed and treated with a number of antiviral drugs. These drugs function by lowering hepatic inflammation, inhibiting the spread of viruses, and averting liver damage. The following antiviral drugs are frequently prescribed to treat hepatitis B:

1. Tenofovir disoproxil fumarate (TDF): TDF is an oral medicine that is a member of the nucleotide analog drug class. It is regarded as one of the most effective hepatitis B antiviral drugs. TDF enhances liver function, lowers hepatic inflammation, and successfully blocks virus multiplication. It has a strong barrier to resistance and is generally well tolerated.

2. Entecavir: Another oral antiviral drug in the nucleoside analogs class is Entecavir. It functions by preventing the reverse transcriptase enzyme, which is required for the replication of viruses. Entecavir works wonders to improve liver function and inhibit viral multiplication. It has a low chance of acquiring resistance and is well-tolerated.

3. Tenofovir alafenamide, or TAF for short, is a more recent formulation of tenofovir that has demonstrated better bone and renal safety than TDF. It effectively inhibits viral reproduction and has a similar antiviral effect. TAF is typically regarded as safe and has

Hepatitis B symptoms can be managed in a number of ways to ease pain, promote liver health, and lower the chance of complications. It is crucial to remember that hepatitis B is a chronic infection and that each individual may experience different symptoms. The following are important elements of symptom management:

1. Medical consultation: Discuss your symptoms with a healthcare provider who has experience treating hepatitis B. Personalized guidance and treatment

choices tailored to your particular situation can be provided by them.

2. Rest and hydration: Make sure you get enough sleep and stay well-hydrated. Hepatitis B frequently causes fatigue, which can be lessened by resting your body and drinking enough water.

3. Medication: To stop the hepatitis B virus (HBV) from replicating in the body, doctors may prescribe antiviral drugs. These drugs can lessen inflammation in the liver, delay the course of the illness, and enhance liver health.

4. Immunizations: Verify that your hepatitis A and hepatitis B shots are current. Since hepatitis A can worsen liver damage in those who already have hepatitis B, immunization is essential to avoiding co-infection.

5. Diet and nutrition: Choose a diet that supports liver function and is well-balanced. Limit your consumption of processed foods, saturated fats, and refined sugars, and stay away from alcohol. Rather, concentrate on eating entire grains, fruits, vegetables, lean meats, and healthy fats.

6. Steer clear of liver toxins: The liver may be harmed by several drugs and chemicals. See your physician before beginning any new pharmaceutical regimen.

6.9 Liver Transplantation: A Life-Saving Treatment for Hepatitis B

A healthy liver from a donor is used in a surgical operation called a liver transplant to replace a damaged or diseased liver. It has become a potentially life-saving treatment for hepatitis B and other liver illnesses. A viral infection called hepatitis B can result in chronic liver damage and serious side effects. Liver transplantation is an effective therapy option if other therapies are not successful or if liver cirrhosis becomes life-threatening. This article will discuss liver transplantation as a treatment for hepatitis B, including its advantages and disadvantages.

The Requirement for Liver Transplantation: When hepatitis B infection advances to advanced stages and causes severe liver damage or cirrhosis, liver transplantation becomes necessary. Hepatocellular carcinoma, or liver failure, can result from a persistent hepatitis B infection.

Pre-transplant evaluation: To ascertain whether a patient is a good candidate for a liver transplant, a comprehensive evaluation is carried out prior to the procedure. A review of the patient's medical history, physical examinations, blood tests, imaging scans, and other diagnostic procedures are all included in this evaluation. It also entails evaluating the patient's general health status, the extent of liver disease, and the existence of liver cancer.

Locating a fit donor for a liver transplant: is a critical step in the transplantation process. A liver transplant is considered when a patient's liver is severely damaged or no longer functions properly. The aim is to replace the damaged liver with a healthy liver from a suitable donor. *Here are the steps involved in locating a fit donor for a liver transplant:*

1. Evaluation: The patient who needs a liver transplant undergoes a thorough evaluation to determine if they are a suitable candidate for the procedure. This evaluation includes medical tests, assessments of liver function, imaging scans, and assessments of overall health.

2. Compatibility: The donor for a liver transplant is usually a deceased person whose liver is suitable for transplantation. Compatibility is determined based on factors such as blood type, size, and weight match between the donor and recipient. The recipient's immune system must also be compatible with the donor organ to minimize the risk of rejection.

3. Waiting list: If a suitable deceased donor is not available immediately, the patient is placed on a waiting list maintained by a national transplant

organization. The allocation of organs is done based on factors such as medical urgency, waiting time, and compatibility.

4. Living donor option: In some cases, a living person can donate a portion of their liver to the patient. This option offers several advantages, including reduced waiting time and better outcomes. The living donor needs to undergo extensive medical and psychological evaluations to ensure their suitability for donation.

5. As a healthcare domain expert, testing the potential donor refers to the process of evaluating an individual's eligibility and suitability for organ or blood donation. This testing is done to ensure the safety and well-being of both the donor and the recipient.

The testing process typically involves several steps:

1. Medical History: The potential donor is required to provide a detailed medical history, including any past illnesses, surgeries, medications, and lifestyle habits. This information helps in assessing the overall health of the donor and identifying any potential risk factors.

2. Physical Examination: A thorough physical examination is conducted to assess the donor's general health, vital signs, and any signs of underlying medical conditions that may disqualify them from donating. This examination may include measurements such as height, weight, blood pressure, and temperature.

3. Laboratory Tests: Various laboratory tests are conducted to evaluate the donor's blood and organ function. These tests may include blood typing, blood

count, liver and kidney function tests, infectious disease screening (HIV, hepatitis, etc.), and genetic testing if necessary. The results of these tests help in determining the donor's overall health and suitability for donation.

4. Psychological Evaluation: In some cases, a psychological evaluation may be conducted to assess the donor's mental health and emotional well-being. This evaluation ensures that the donor understands the risks and responsibilities associated with the donation process and is capable of providing informed consent.

5. Compatibility Testing: For organ transplantation, further compatibility testing is conducted between the donor and recipient.

As a healthcare domain expert, here are the steps involved in locating a fit donor for a liver transplant:

1. Referral and Evaluation: The first step is for the patient in need of a liver transplant to be referred to a transplant center. The patient then undergoes a comprehensive evaluation to determine whether they are suitable candidates for a liver transplant.

2. Blood Typing and Compatibility Testing: The patient's blood type is determined, and compatibility testing is done to identify potential matches. This includes testing for human leukocyte antigens (HLAs) to assess immune compatibility.

3. Waitlisting: If the patient is deemed eligible, they are placed on a national organ transplant waiting list. The allocation of organs is based on factors such as medical urgency, blood type, body size, and time spent on the waiting list.

4. Donor Identification: Donor identification involves identifying deceased donors who are a suitable match for the patient. This is done by evaluating factors such as blood type, size, and medical compatibility.

5. Organ Offer: If a potential donor is identified, the transplant center receives an offer for the organ. A thorough evaluation of the donor's medical history and liver function is conducted to ensure its suitability for transplantation.

6. Organ Acceptance: The transplant team reviews the donor information and determines whether to accept the organ for the patient. Factors evaluated include the donor's age, cause of death, medical conditions, and overall organ quality.

7. Transplant Procedure: If the organ is

Certainly! A liver transplant is a complex surgical procedure that involves replacing a diseased or damaged liver with a healthy liver from a donor. Here is a simplified explanation of the procedure:

1. Evaluation: The first step is a thorough evaluation to determine if a patient is a suitable candidate for a liver transplant. This evaluation includes medical tests, imaging scans, and consultations with a transplant team that consists of hepatologists (liver specialists), surgeons, anesthesiologists, and other healthcare professionals.

2. Waiting List: If the patient meets the criteria for a liver transplant, they are placed on a waiting list for a suitable donor liver. The allocation of donor livers is based on factors like blood type, severity of illness, and time spent on the waiting list.

3. Preoperative Preparation: Once a suitable donor liver becomes available, the patient is admitted to the hospital and prepared for surgery. This includes blood tests, imaging scans, and other preoperative procedures to ensure the patient is in optimal condition for the transplant.

4. Anesthesia and Incision: The patient is given general anesthesia, and the surgeon makes an incision in the abdomen to access the liver.

5. Dissection and Preparation: The surgeon carefully dissects and removes the patient's diseased liver, taking care to preserve important blood vessels and bile ducts. The bile ducts and blood vessels of the donor liver are also dissected and prepared for connection.

6. Implantation: The healthy donor liver is carefully implanted.

Implantation of a healthy donor liver, also known as liver transplantation, is a surgical procedure performed to replace a diseased or damaged liver with a healthy liver from a living or deceased donor. This procedure is typically recommended for patients with end-stage liver disease, acute liver failure, or certain liver cancers.

The implantation process involves several steps:

1. Donor Evaluation: For a living donor transplantation, potential donors undergo a thorough evaluation to ensure they are healthy and suitable for donation. This includes medical tests, imaging studies, and psychological assessments. In the case of deceased donor transplantation, the liver is procured from a deceased individual who has previously consented to organ donation.

2. Organ Procurement: In deceased donor transplantation, the liver is procured from the donor following their death. The liver is removed from the donor's body while preserving its blood vessels, bile ducts, and other vital structures.

3. Recipient Preparation: The recipient is prepared for surgery, which includes preoperative tests, blood matching, and placement on the waiting list for a suitable donor liver. The recipient may be required to follow a specific diet, take medications, and manage their condition while waiting for a transplant.

4. Implantation: The recipient is brought to the operating room, and anesthesia is administered. The surgeon makes an incision and carefully removes the recipient's damaged liver. The blood vessels and bile

ducts are meticulously connected to the healthy donor liver.

6.10 Hepatitis B symptoms

Hepatitis B symptoms can be managed in a number of ways to ease pain, promote liver health, and lower the chance of complications. It is crucial to remember that hepatitis B is a chronic infection and that each individual may experience different symptoms. The following are important elements of symptom management:

1. Medical consultation: Discuss your symptoms with a healthcare provider who has experience treating hepatitis B. Personalized guidance and treatment solutions tailored to your particular situation can be offered by them.

2. Rest and hydration: Make sure you get enough sleep and stay well-hydrated. Hepatitis B frequently causes fatigue, which can be lessened by resting your body and drinking enough water.

3. Medication: To stop the hepatitis B virus (HBV) from replicating in the body, doctors may prescribe antiviral drugs. These drugs can lessen inflammation in the liver, delay the course of the illness, and enhance liver health.

4. Immunizations: Verify that your hepatitis A and hepatitis B shots are current. Vaccination is essential in preventing co-infection because hepatitis A can exacerbate liver damage in those who already have hepatitis B.

5. Diet and nutrition: Choose a diet that supports liver function and is well-balanced. Limit your consumption

of processed foods, saturated fats, and refined sugars, and stay away from alcohol. Rather, concentrate on eating entire grains, fruits, vegetables, lean meats, and healthy fats.

6. Steer clear of liver toxins: The liver may be harmed by several drugs and chemicals. See your physician before beginning any new pharmaceutical regimen.

6.11 Managing Hepatitis B

Although having Hepatitis B might be difficult, a happy life can be had with the right information, resources, and way of life. When managing Hepatitis B, keep the following considerations in mind:

1. Education and Awareness: It's critical to spread knowledge about Hepatitis B to both you and those in your vicinity. Recognize the signs, symptoms, and possible consequences of the infection. With this knowledge, you can stop the infection from spreading and make well-informed decisions regarding your health.

2. Routine Medical Monitoring: Routine examinations by a physician with expertise in Hepatitis B are crucial. They can keep an eye on the condition of your liver, monitor the virus's activity, and, if necessary, recommend the right course of action.

3. Medication and Treatment: Antiviral drugs may be recommended to decrease the virus's reproduction and reduce the risk of liver damage, depending on the severity of the infection. Pay close attention to what

your doctor tells you, and take your prescription drugs on a regular basis.

4. Vaccination: To stop the spread of the disease, make sure your family members and close friends have had the Hepatitis B vaccine. In terms of preventing new infections, the Hepatitis B vaccine is both safe and effective.

5. Healthy Lifestyle: Changing to a healthier lifestyle will make a big difference in your general wellbeing. Eat a healthy, balanced diet, do regular exercise, abstain from alcohol, and quit smoking. Making these lifestyle changes can help maintain the health of your liver and lower the likelihood of developing new issues.

6. Emotional Support: Living with a chronic condition like Hepatitis B may cause emotional stress. Seek support from friends and family.

CHAPTER SEVEN

Living with Hepatitis B can be challenging, but with proper knowledge, support, and lifestyle choices, it is possible to lead a fulfilling life. Here are some key points to consider when living with Hepatitis B:

1. Education and Awareness: It is crucial to educate yourself and those around you about Hepatitis B. Understand how the virus is transmitted, its symptoms, and potential complications. This knowledge will help you make informed decisions about your health and prevent the spread of the virus.

2. Regular Medical Monitoring: Regular check-ups with a healthcare professional specializing in Hepatitis B are essential. They can monitor your liver's health, track the virus's

activity, and prescribe appropriate treatments if necessary.

3. Medication and Treatment: Depending on the severity of the infection, antiviral medications may be prescribed to suppress the replication of the virus and lower the risk of liver damage. Follow your healthcare provider's instructions carefully, and take the prescribed medications regularly.

4. Vaccination: Make sure your loved ones and close contacts are vaccinated against Hepatitis B to prevent transmission. The Hepatitis B vaccine is safe and effective in preventing new infections.

5. Healthy Lifestyle: Adopting a healthy lifestyle can significantly improve your overall well-being. Maintain a balanced diet, exercise

regularly, and avoid alcohol and tobacco. These lifestyle choices can help keep your liver healthy and reduce the risk of further complications.

6. Emotional Support: Living with a chronic condition like Hepatitis B may cause emotional stress. Seek support from friends and family.

Supportive care plays a crucial role in the management of hepatitis B, a viral infection that affects the liver. While specific antiviral treatment may be necessary for certain cases, supportive care focuses on alleviating symptoms, minimizing liver damage, and promoting overall well-being. *Here are some important aspects of supportive care for hepatitis B:*

1. Lifestyle modifications: Adopting a healthy lifestyle is vital to supporting liver health. This

includes maintaining a balanced diet, avoiding alcohol and harmful substances, and engaging in regular exercise. A nutritious diet can help boost the immune system and improve liver function.

2. Medications: Certain medications may be prescribed to manage the symptoms of hepatitis B. These can include antiviral drugs to suppress viral replication as well as medications to manage symptoms such as nausea, fatigue, and muscle aches.

3. Regular monitoring: It is essential to regularly monitor liver function through blood tests to assess the severity of hepatitis B and identify any signs of liver damage. This allows healthcare providers to adjust treatment plans accordingly.

4. Vaccinations: Vaccinations against hepatitis A and B are recommended for individuals with hepatitis B, as co-infection can cause more severe liver damage.

5. Emotional support: Living with a chronic condition like hepatitis B can have a significant impact on mental health. It is important to seek emotional support from healthcare professionals, support groups, or therapists who specialize in chronic illnesses.

6. Education and prevention: educating oneself and others about hepatitis B transmission, prevention methods, and the importance

7.3 Nurturing Emotional Well-Being for Individuals Living with Hepatitis B

Living with hepatitis B can present unique challenges that can impact not only your physical health but also your emotional well-being. It is essential to prioritize your mental and emotional health to lead a fulfilling life despite the diagnosis. *Here in this book will provide helpful strategies and support for individuals living with hepatitis B to nurture their emotional well-being.*

Seek Support: Living with hepatitis B can feel isolating, but remember that you are not alone. Seek support from friends, family, or support groups that focus on hepatitis B. Connecting with others who understand your journey can provide valuable emotional support and a sense of belonging.

Educate Yourself: Empower yourself by learning more about hepatitis B. Understand the facts, treatment options, and ways to manage the condition. By becoming knowledgeable about your condition, you can better advocate for yourself and reduce feelings of uncertainty or anxiety.

Practice Self-Care: Prioritize self-care to promote emotional well-being. Engage in activities you enjoy, such as hobbies, exercise, or meditation. Take time to relax, rest, and recharge. Eating a balanced diet, getting enough sleep, and avoiding excessive alcohol or drug use are also important for overall well-being.

Communicate Openly: Effective communication is vital for emotional well-being. Talk openly with your healthcare team about any concerns or questions you may have.

conccusion

In the book "Hepatitis B: A Journey Towards Understanding and Prevention," we embark on a comprehensive exploration of one of the world's most prevalent and persistent infectious diseases. Hepatitis B is a viral infection that affects millions of people worldwide, with serious implications for public health. However, through this enlightening and informative guide, we aim to provide readers with a deeper understanding of this condition, its causes, symptoms, treatment options, and, most importantly, the preventive measures that can be taken to combat its spread.

In this book, we delve into the basics of hepatitis B, understanding its viral nature, modes of transmission, and the various factors that contribute to its prevalence. We explore the global impact of hepatitis B, highlighting the regions most affected and shedding light on the burden it places on individuals, families, and healthcare systems. Here, we explore the diverse spectrum of symptoms associated with hepatitis B, from mild flu-like symptoms to more severe manifestations such as jaundice and liver failure. We discuss the importance of early diagnosis as well as the diagnostic tests available to identify hepatitis B infection, including blood tests and imaging techniques. In this chapter, we provide an overview of the available treatment options for hepatitis B. It delves into the complex topic of hepatitis B, focusing specifically on asymptomatic infections and the methods used to diagnose and monitor the disease. It explains what asymptomatic infection means in the context of hepatitis B, highlighting the significance of individuals who carry the virus but do not exhibit any symptoms. It emphasizes the importance of detecting and managing these cases to prevent transmission and reduce the risk of complications.

Subsequently, the book provides a comprehensive overview of the various diagnostic methods available for hepatitis B. It explores both serological tests and molecular assays, discussing their strengths, limitations, and appropriate clinical applications. The significance of an accurate diagnosis in determining disease progression and guiding treatment decisions is emphasized throughout. Furthermore, the book discusses the different phases of hepatitis B infection, including acute, chronic, and resolved infections. It explores the role of serological markers, such as HBsAg, anti-HBs, and anti-HBc, in monitoring disease progression and assessing treatment efficacy. Additionally, it highlights the importance of regular monitoring and surveillance of patients with chronic hepatitis B to detect disease reactivation, evaluate liver function, and identify potential complications, such as hepatocellular carcinoma. It emphasizes the need for a multidisciplinary approach involving healthcare professionals from various specialties to ensure the comprehensive management of

The book also focuses on the importance of regular monitoring and screening for individuals living with Hepatitis B. The book provides an overview of Hepatitis B, its transmission methods, and the potential risks associated with the virus. It emphasizes the significance of routine screening to detect the virus at an early stage, which is crucial for effective management and prevention of complications. It also discusses various screening methods available, such as blood tests and serological markers, and their effectiveness in detecting hepatitis B infection. It emphasizes the need for healthcare professionals to stay updated on the latest screening guidelines and recommendations.

Furthermore, the book highlights the significance of regular monitoring for individuals with chronic hepatitis B. It discusses the various parameters that should be monitored, including liver function tests, viral load, and liver imaging. The book emphasizes the importance of individualized monitoring plans based on the patient's specific needs and risk factors. It focuses on the emotional and psychological impact of hepatitis B on individuals living with the virus. The book emphasizes the need for comprehensive care that addresses not only the physical health but also the emotional well-being of these individuals. It also explores the various emotional challenges faced by individuals living with Hepatitis B, such as stigma, fear, and anxiety. It discusses the importance of healthcare professionals providing a supportive and non-judgmental environment to foster emotional well-being.

www.ingramcontent.com/pod-product-compliance
Lightning Source LLC
Chambersburg PA
CBHW072216290526
45794CB00004B/1765